First Aid
for
Sports Injuries

Third Edition

Stanley H. Inkelis. M.D.
Professor of Pediatrics &
Emergency Medicine
UCLA School of Medicine

Eric Golanty, Ph.D.
Emeritus Professor of Health,
Wellness, & Physical Education
Las Positas College

First Aid for Sports Injuries

Many thanks to principal reviewer Erin Rosenberg, M.S., former instructor, Department of Athletic Training and Assistant Director, Entry-level Athletic Training Programs at Ohio University.

ISBN: 0-9842644-1-8
ISBN-13: 978-0-9842644-1-4

This book and its associated digital editions, mobile application, and Web site are intended to provide accurate information for educational purposes and are not intended to replace competent medical advice and care offered by a physician or other health professional.

All information is presented for educational purposes only, not as medical advice, and presented "as is" without warranty or guarantee of any kind. Readers are cautioned not to rely on this information as medical advice and to consult a qualified medical professional for their specific needs.

No responsibility or liability is assumed by the authors or publisher for any injury, damage, or financial loss sustained to persons or property from the use of this information, personal or otherwise, either directly or indirectly. While every effort has been made to ensure reliability and accuracy of the information within, all liability, negligence or otherwise, from any use, misuse or abuse of the operation of any methods, strategies, instructions or ideas contained in the material herein, is the sole responsibility of the reader or application-user.

The information in this book, its associated digital editions, Web site, and mobile applications has not been evaluated by the Federal Trade Commission, Food and Drug Administration, or any other government agency and it is not intended to diagnose, treat, cure, or prevent any disease.

First Aid for Sports Injuries Digital Edition
for
Smart Phones and Tablets

First Aid
for
Sports
Injuries

Fast access to helpful information when someone is injured at practice, during competition, working out, and at recreational play.

More info:
***First Aid for Sports Injuries* Web site**
http://ergo84.com/fa/

CONTENTS

ATTENDING TO COMMON SPORTS INJURIES

CONTENTS

SPORTS INJURY BASICS

First Aid for Sports Injuries

PREFACE

In the best cases, every work out, practice, and competition
would have on hand a professional who is trained or certified to
respond to sports injuries. Since that is not always the case,
coaches, parents, and athletes are left to attend to sports injuries
as best as they can on their own. For such situations, we offer
the information in this book so that an injury can receive at least
some attention until competent medical care is obtained.

To best utilize this book:

1. Familiarize yourself with the book's contents so you will
know what kind of information it offers. Tag these pages so
you can get to them quickly:
- Unconsciousness, page 2
- Cardiopulmonary Resuscitation (CPR), page 3
- Breathing Problem, page 4
- Serious Bleeding, page 6
- Head and Neck Injury, page 13

2. Practice wrapping an elastic wrap ("Ace" bandage). Video
directions at http://www.ergo84.com/fa/wrapping.html

3. Practice CPR and Rescue Breathing. Video directions at
http://www.ergo84.com/fa/breathe.html

4. Obtain a sports injury first aid kit. Links and info at
http://www.ergo84.com/fa/fakits.html

5. Familiarize yourself with sports injury prevention strategies
as described at http:///www.ergo84.com/fa/prevent.html

6. If you are a coach, designate someone to be familiar with
responding to an injury as you may be too busy during practice
or a competition to attend to it yourself.

7. Understand that this book is educational and not intended to
be a substitute for competent medical care. References on page
40.

Stan Inkelis and Eric Golanty, Authors

IMMEDIATE FIRST AID -- R.I.C.E.

Rest - Ice - Compression - Elevation

REST: Rest and immobilize the injured region to retard swelling and internal bleeding.

ICE: Cover the injured region with a cold pack, crushed ice or ice cubes in a towel, an ice bag, or frozen peas for 10-30 minutes. DO NOT put ice on bare skin or directly over a nerve. Remove ice for 15 minutes; re-ice for 15-30 minutes over the span of three hours.

COMPRESSION: Wrap the injured region in an elastic ("Ace") bandage to retard swelling (video link below). Be sure to overlap the elastic bandage by one-half to one-third of its width each time you go around (i.e., leave no spaces or holes). Remove the wrap if compression increases pain, the skin turns pale or blue, or there is numbness, tingling, or a loss of sensation.

ELEVATION: Elevate the injured region (particularly a limb) to control swelling and internal bleeding.

Video: How to wrap an elastic bandage
http://www.ergo84.com/fa/wrapping.html

References on page 40

UNCONSCIOUSNESS

Call for professional help immediately.

1. Try to awaken the vicim by tapping him or her vigorously and shouting, "Are you all right!?"

2. No response? Check if the person is breathing (Is the chest/stomach moving? Is faint air escaping the mouth?).

3. If not breathing, lay the victim flat on her or his back. If necessary, roll the victim over, moving the head and body simultaneously to avoid worsening a possible neck injury.

4. Loosen clothing around the head and chest.

5. Remove foreign material from the victim's mouth:
   • Hold the victim's mouth open with your hand and depress the tongue with your thumb.
   • Use your index finger on the other hand like a hook to sweep the victim's mouth clear.

6. Continue to monitor heart beat and breathing every few minutes until EMS or other health professional arrives.

7. DO NOT
   • give an unconscious person any food or drink.
   • leave the person alone.
   • place a pillow under the head of an unconscious person.
   • slap or splash water on the face to try to revive an unconscious person.

References on page 40

First Aid for Sports Injuries

CPR (*Cardiopulmonary Resuscitation*)

CPR is carried out on someone who has stopped breathing or whose heart has stopped.

Immediate Attention (age > 8 years)

1. FIRST! Check for consciousness. Tap on the shoulder and shout,"Are you all right!?" DO NOT SHAKE in case of damage to the spinal cord. Have someone call 911.

Untrained at CPR:
2. Lay the victim flat on the back. If necessary, roll the victim over, moving head and body simultaneously to avoid worsening a possible neck injury.

3. Kneel next to the victim's neck and shoulders.

4. Place the heel of your hand over the center of the victim's chest, between the nipples. Place your other hand on top of the first hand. Lock your elbows straight. Position your shoulders directly above your hands.

5. Push down using your upper body weight (not just your arms); compress the chest about two inches.

6. Deliver 100 chest compressions per minute until EMS arrive.

Trained at CPR:
2. As #1 above except:
• Deliver 30 chest compressions (as above).
• Administer Rescue Breathing (see pages 4-5)

CPR on a Child (Age 1-8)
2. As #1 above except:
• Use only one hand to perform compressions.
• Use cycles of 30 compression/2 breaths until EMS arrive.

Video: http://www.ergo84.com/fa/cpr.html

References on page 40

3

BREATHING PROBLEM

FIRST! Check for consciousness. Tap on the shoulder and shout, "Are you all right!?"   DO NOT SHAKE in case of damage to the spinal cord. No response, call 911.

General Rules

1. If breathing has stopped or has become very faint, open the victim's airway and begin rescue breathing (video link below).

2. Immediately have someone else summon professional help. If you are alone, shout or phone for help. Do not leave the victim alone under any circumstances.

3. NEAR-DROWNING: DO NOT give rescue breathing if the victim can breathe without assistance, even though coughing, sputtering, choking, or vomiting.

Opening the Airway

1. If no head or neck injury is apparent, tip the victim's head back by placing the palm of your hand on the forehead and simultaneously lifting up on the chin with two fingers of your other hand.

2. Listen for breath sounds by placing your ear close to the victim's mouth for about 10 seconds. Watch for movement of the chest or stomach.

3. Begin rescue breathing immediately (see adjacent page) if breathing is very faint or if there is doubt that the victim is breathing.

Video: http://www.ergo84.com/fa/cpr.html

References on page 40

4

First Aid for Sports Injuries

Mouth-to Mouth Rescue Breathing (age > 8 years)

1. Place your hand on the victim's forehead, pinch the nose closed with your fingers while keeping the airway open.

2. Take a deep breath. Place your mouth over the victim's mouth and blow air into him or her until you see the chest rise. Repeat quickly 4 times without the victim's lungs deflating between breaths.

3. Raise your head and watch for movement of the victim's chest and listen for air escaping from the nose and mouth. If the chest falls or you can hear air escaping, rescue breathing is proceeding. If not, the airway may be blocked or the victim's body or head position may need correcting.

4. Repeat giving one breath every 5 seconds (count 1-1000, 2-1000 etc.).

Rescue Breathing for Children 2-8 years

Perform steps as above except...

• Look for foreign material in the mouth before sweeping the mouth with a finger to avoid pushing material into the throat. Remove any foreign material with a sweep of the finger.

• Deliver 4 gentle breaths rapidly without allowing the child's lungs to deflate entirely between breaths. Blow in only the amount needed to inflate the lungs; gentle puffs are often sufficient.

• Repeat rescue breathing every 3-4 seconds (15-20 breaths/minute). The child's chest should rise and fall with rescue breathing. If not, check for airway obstruction or the need to reposition the body or head.

References on Page 40

BLEEDING (SERIOUS)

STOP! the bleeding with direct pressure on the wound. Wear latex gloves to prevent transmission of HIV and other infections. Remain calm and in control. Reassure the bleeding person using a calm, firm voice.

If the injury is to the head, neck, abdomen, or leg, do not move the person or you may make things worse. Otherwise, lay the person down and cover the person with a jacket or blanket.

Immediate Attention

1. With a sterile gauze pad, clean handkerchief, or gloved hand if necessary, apply firm, steady pressure over the wound.

2. If a dressing becomes soaked with blood, apply another dressing. Do not remove the original dressing. Do not peek at the wound to see if the bleeding has stopped.

3. Elevate an injured hand, arm, leg, or foot above the level of the heart to slow blood loss.

4. Apply gentle pressure to a scalp wound.

5. Apply a tourniquet ONLY if direct pressure is unsuccessful at stopping bleeding and only for a maximum of 30 minutes.

6. Do not probe a wound to seek or remove an embedded object.

Consult a physician IF...

• bleeding cannot be controlled even with a tourniquet.
• foreign material cannot be removed from the wound.
• bleeding is from the ear or scalp.
• there is coughing or vomiting blood.
• bleeding is from the chest or abdomen (sign of possible internal bleeding).
• a tetanus shot has not been received in the prior 5 years.

References on Page 40

CUT (*Laceration*)

Immediate Attention

1. Wear latex gloves to prevent transmission of HIV and other infections. Remain calm and in control. Reassure the bleeding person using a calm, firm voice.

2. Cleanse the wound with soap and warm water from a tap, a plastic squeeze bottle, or a rubber bulb to rinse away dirt and particles. Antiseptic is not required but may be used if desired.

Consult a physician IF...

- a serious cut is on the face, scalp, chest, abdomen, back, or extremities.
- the cut is gaping or deep; profuse bleeding may require stitches to close the wound.
- the cut is from a human or animal bite.
- blood spurts forcefully from the wound.
- fat protrudes from the wound.
- there is doubt that all foreign matter has been removed from the wound.
- signs of infection occur (pus, redness, swelling, fever).
- a tetanus shot has not been received in the prior 5 years.

References on Page 40

NOSEBLEED

Wear latex gloves to prevent transmission of HIV and other infections. Remain calm and in control. Reassure the bleeding person using a calm, firm voice.

Immediate Attention

1. The person should sit with the head tilted slightly forward to prevent blood from entering the breathing apparatus or throat.

2. The person should remain quiet and still.

3. Apply pressure to close the bleeding nostril, pinch both nostrils for 5-10 minutes, or place a rolled gauze pad under the lip against the gum.

4. Apply ice or cold pack to the nose and face.

5. If direct pressure does not work, insert a small sterile gauze into the bleeding nostril and pinch closed.

6. Do not pick or blow the nose and do not bend down for several hours after the bleeding stops.

Consult a physician IF...

- bleeding persists for more than 10 minutes.
- the nosebleed was due to a fall or blow to the face or head.
- nosebleeds are recurrent.
- other bruises are evident.
- the person bruises easily or bleeds easily and profusely.

References on Page 41

PUNCTURE

Wear latex gloves to prevent transmission of HIV and other infections. Remain calm and in control. Reassure the bleeding person using a calm, firm voice.

Immediate Attention

1. Remove foreign objects in the skin with tweezers or a sterilized (with flame or alcohol pad) sewing needle.

2. Objects lodged deep in the skin should be removed by a health care professional.

Minor Punctures

1. Let the wound bleed for a few minutes to facilitate removal of dirt, particles, and bacteria from the wound.

2. Wash the wound with soap and warm water. Antiseptic, while unnecessary, may be applied if desired.

3. Dress the wound with a sterile adhesive strip or gauze bandage secured with adhesive or surgical tape.

4. Remove the dressing and cleanse the wound 4-5 times a day for 4-5 days.

Consult a physician IF...

- the wound is on the face, trunk, hand, foot, or a joint.
- bleeding is severe and will not stop.
- numbness or a tingling sensation occurs.
- blood spurts forcefully from the wound.
- the wound was sustained through a shoe or other clothing.
- there is doubt that all foreign matter has been removed from the wound.
- signs of infection occur (pus, redness, swelling, fever).
- a tetanus shot has not been received in the prior 5 years.

References on Page 40

First Aid for Sports Injuries

SCRAPE (*Abrasion*)

Wear latex gloves to prevent transmission of HIV and other infections. Remain calm and in control. Reassure the bleeding person using a calm, firm voice.

Immediate Attention

1. Cleanse the wound with soap and warm water from a tap, a plastic squeeze bottle, or rubber bulb to rinse away dirt and particles. Antiseptic is not required but may be used if desired.

2. Remove debris remaining after washing with a washcloth or soft brush.

3. Do not bandage the wound unless bleeding persists and then only to stop the bleeding.

4. If returning to play, cover any wound to protect the athlete and others.

Consult a physician IF...

- a serious wound is on the face, scalp, chest, abdomen, back, or extremities.
- the wound is jagged, gaping, or deep.
- the cut is over a joint.
- the wound is from a human or animal bite.
- blood spurts forcefully from the wound.
- fat protrudes from the wound.
- there is doubt that all foreign matter has been removed from the wound.
- signs of infection occur (pus, redness, swelling, fever).
- a tetanus shot has not been received in the prior 5 years.

DENTAL INJURIES

Injuries to the mouth and teeth occur most often from direct blows to the face, which result in bleeding, displacement of a tooth, chipped, broken or knocked out teeth, and fractures of the jaw or other facial bones.

Immediate Attention

Tooth/Mouth Bleeding

1. Put on gloves. Put direct finger pressure with sterile gauze over the area of bleeding.

Loose/Damaged Teeth

1. Loose Tooth: If pushed back, pulled forward, or hanging down, gently push the tooth back into its normal position. See a dentist ASAP.

2. Missing Tooth: Find the tooth; save it in whole milk. See a dentist or physician within 30 minutes to have the tooth put back in place.

3. Broken Tooth: Save the broken portion. Follow directions in #2 above.

Consult a physician IF...

- a tooth is broken or knocked out.
- a tooth is pushed into the gum (looks short).
- a facial bone is fractured.

References on Page 41

11

EYE INJURIES

Immediate Attention

Eye Bruise ("Black Eye")

1. Apply ice or a cold pack as soon as possible.

Foreign Object in the Eye

1. Do not rub the eye.

2. Do not attempt to remove the object with fingers, toothpick, or any other object.

3. Lower eye: Gently pull down the lower eyelid. An object on the inner surface may be removed with the edge of a sterile gauze bandage or the edge of a clean handkerchief.

4. Upper eye: Gently pull the upper eyelid over the lower eyelid with the person looking down. The resultant tears may dislodge the object onto the lower eyelid, thereby facilitating removal.

Sunlight Damage ("Snow Blindness")

1. Cover the eyes with patches or light-proof bandages for 24 hours.

2. If desired, take aspirin or acetaminophen for pain (see pg 23).

Consult a physician IF...

• the eye has been cut or punctured. Shield the eye with the bottom of a paper cup taped to the face.
• vision is impaired, the eye has sustained a direct blow, or eye movement is restricted.
• an object cannot be removed, is embedded in the surface of the eye, or has penetrated the eye. Cover both eyes with patches or gauze bandages secured with tape to reduce eye movement.
• snow blindness.

References on Page 41

HEAD AND NECK INJURIES

Immediate Attention

1. Any complaint of head or neck pain is reason to stop athletic activity.

2. Suspect a neck injury if there is pain or tenderness in the neck or weakness in the extremities, the person behaves abnormally, is drowsy, vomits more than once, or loses consciousness, even briefly.

3. Do not move the injured person. The injured person should not stand or sit. Keep the head in a neutral position.

4. If the injured person is not breathing, open the airway and give rescue breathing. Do not move the person's head or neck while giving rescue breathing.

5. If the injured person must be turned over to administer rescue breathing, control the head and neck and move the person simultaneously with the entire body.

6. If the injured person can be transported, move her or him with a backboard, being careful to move the head and neck with the rest of the body.

7. Control bleeding from scalp or face by direct pressure.

8. If possible, do not remove headgear. Use bolt cutters to remove a face guard or a helmet if CPR is to be administered.

Consult a physician IF...

- there is severe facial or head bleeding.
- the person stops breathing.
- a severe head or neck injury us suspected even if there are no symptoms.

References on Page 41

13

GENITAL INJURY

Immediate Attention

1. Significant bleeding from a cut: apply pressure as with any bleeding injury

2. Bleeding from the urethra: delay urination until a physician is consulted.

Testicular Injury

- Lie on the back with the legs bent.
- Take slow, steady, deep breaths.
- If the injury is significant, apply ice or a cold pack.
- Elevate scrotum on several rolled towels placed between the legs.
- Rest until able to walk; resume activity when ready.

Vulvar Injury

- Apply ice or a cold pack to contusions of the vulva or vagina.
- Rest until able to walk; resume activity when ready.

Consult a physician IF...

- scrotum pain persists for more than one hour.
- there is swelling or blood in the scrotum.
- one or both testes cannot be located in the scrotum.
- there is pain on urination, urination is not possible, or there is blood in the urine.
- there is bleeding from the urethra.
- there is a laceration of the penis, scrotum, vulva, or vagina.
- there is vaginal bleeding not associated with menstruation.
- there is any penetrating injury to the genitalia.
- a female experiences abdominal pain after injury.

References on Page 41

COLD STRESS (*Hypothermia*)

Overexposure to cold, windy, wet weather may produce abnormally low body temperature. Symptoms include shivering, muscle weakness, numbness, drowsiness, and occasionally unconsciousness.

Immediate Attention

1. Give rescue breathing if necessary.

2. Remove the victim from the cold environment; handle gently; protect the victim from wind.

3. Keep the victim still.

4. Replace wet, cold clothing with warm.

5. Rewarm the victim by immersing in warm (105-110 F degree) water, wrapping in warm blankets, or providing skin-to-skin contact with a warm person.

6. Do not give alcohol to "warm up."

Consult a physician immediately as hypothermia can be fatal.

References on Page 42

FROSTBITE

Frostbite is frozen body tissue with ice crystals in body fluids. The skin is white or grayish-yellow. It can be painful at first but pain diminishes as tissues freeze.

Immediate Attention

1. Rewarm the person by immersing in warm (105-110 F degree) water, wrapping in warm blankets, or providing skin-to-skin contact with a warm person.

2. Do not rewarm a frostbitten region if further exposure to cold and refreezing are likely.

3. Do no rub or massage the affected region.

4. Separate frostbitten fingers and toes with sterile gauze pads. Fingers can be exercised but no walking on frostbitten feet.

Consult a physician immediately.

References on Page 42

HEAT STRESS (*Hyperthermia*)

Heat stress results from elevated body temperature generally from exertion in a hot, humid climate and/or from wearing clothes that trap body heat even in a cold environment. Signs of heat stress include hot, dry skin, nausea, vomiting, headaches, fainting, dizziness, seizures, and unconsciousness.

Heat Cramps

1. Stop activity.

2. Replace body fluids and minerals by drinking water, replacement fluids, or dilute 100% fruit juice.

3. Massage and stretch cramping muscles. Applying cold packs may also help.

4. Rest and cool the body to normal before resuming activity.

Heat Exhaustion

Signs generally include cool, moist skin, headache, feeling faint or dizzy, heavy sweating, feeling tired and weak, fast heart rate, muscle cramps, nausea, and vision changes.

1. Stop activity. Move to a cooler, shady area.

2. Recline and elevate the legs 12-18 inches.

3. Replace body fluids and minerals by drinking water, replacement fluids, or dilute 100% fruit juice.

4. Cool with wet cloths or cold packs.

5. Rest several days before resuming activity.

Consult a physician immediately

References on Page 42

HEAT STROKE

Signs (not all may be evident): Body temperature >104 F (40 C); flushed skin; rapid, shallow breathing; racing heart rate; headache; muscle cramps or weakness; vision changes; seizures; unconsciousness.

1. ASAP! (within 30 minutes), immerse in cold water to reduce body temperature below 102 degrees F. Otherwise, pour water over the body, apply ice packs to the chest, abdomen, forehead, neck, and legs. If an immersion tub is unavailable do not send the victim to a hospital until core temperature is lowered.

2. If conscious, give water, sports replacement fluids, or dilute 100% fruit juice.

Summon emergency medical services immediately.

Consult a physician immediately.

References on Page 42

BROKEN BONE (*Fracture*)

Signs of a broken bone include having heard a snap or cracking sound in the injured region, limb deformation, or a part of a bone protruding through the skin. Even if there are no obvious signs of a break, the area around a fracture is likely to be tender and swollen.

Immediate Attention

1. Stop any bleeding. Apply a cold pack or ice to limit swelling.

2. Do not move, bend, or straighten the injured body part.

3. Do not try to realign a bone break or reposition a broken bone protruding through the skin.

4. Immobilize a fracture with a splint when professional help is not available.
• fractured leg: tie or tape the injured limb to the noninjured limb.
• fractured arm, elbow bent: tie or tape to the chest.
• fractured arm, elbow straight: tie or tape to the side.
• tie or pin a pillow as a splint.
• cut up and pad a cardboard box for a 3-sided emergency splint.

Consult a physician IF...

• a broken bone is suspected even if not obvious.
• the victim's extremities are numb or bluish.

References on Page 42

MUSCLE CRAMP

A muscle cramp is a painful, extended, involuntary contraction of a muscle.

Immediate Attention

1. Firmly grasp the affected muscle and gradually stretch it until the cramp is relieved.

2. Gently massage the muscle. Icing the muscle may also help.

3. Take slow, deep breaths. Imagine the air going in and out of the body through the cramping muscle instead of the lungs.

4. Replace lost body fluids and minerals with water, replacement fluid, or dilute 100% juice.

5. If desired, take acetaminophen or ibuprofen for pain (see page 23).

Consult a physician IF...

- a cramp cannot be relieved.
- cramping is severe.
- muscle cramps occur frequently.
- cramps are not related to an obvious cause such as exercise.

References on Page 42

MUSCLE PULL (*Strain*)

Pulling (straining) a muscle is due to overstretching or tearing some or all of the fibers in a muscle or its tendon.

Immediate Attention

1. Apply ice or a cold pack as soon as possible.

2. Wrap the muscle with an elastic bandage to control swelling.

3. Elevate the injured region.

4. Take two acetaminophen or ibuprofen for pain (see page 23).

5. Pain is a signal to stop athletic activity.

Consult a physician IF...

• there is near or complete loss of function in the injured region.
• pain and/or swelling continue for more than one week.

References on Page 42

SPRAIN

Sprain results from overstretching or tearing a ligament generally causing instability of a joint or misalignment of bones in a joint (*dislocation*).

Immediate Attention

1. Apply ice or a cold pack as soon as possible and continue cold treatment 4 times a day for 10-15 minutes each time during the first 24-72 hours.

2. Rest and wrap with an elastic bandage to control swelling and soreness.

3. Elevate the injured region.

4. Avoid weight-bearing in the injured region until pain diminishes and normal range of motion returns.

5. Take acetaminophen or ibuprofen to reduce pain (see page 23).

6. Pain is a signal to stop athletic activity.

Consult a physician IF...

• there is near or complete loss of function in the injured region.
• the injury causes any anatomical deformities.
• pain and/or swelling persist longer than two days.
• there is significant redness or swelling around the injury.
• the injured athlete is a child or adolescent.
• a broken bone is suspected.

References on Page 43

PAIN

Sports injury pain is caused by fluid and substances released from damaged tissue. Pain signals that activity should stop; it is not a sign of weakness or lack of desire.

Over-the-Counter Pain Medications for Sports Injuries
• Acetaminophen ("Tylenol")
• Aspirin
• Ibuprofen ("Advil" or "Motrin")
• Naproxen ("Aleve" or "Naprosyn")

Adult Dose
• *Acetaminophen*: not more than 1 gram (1000 mg) per dose or 4 grams (4000 mg) per day. Taking more risks liver damage.
• *Aspirin*: two, 325 mg tablets every 4 hours; not more than 5 times per day.
• *Ibuprofen*: 200mg-400 mg every 4-6 hours; take with food.
• *Naproxen*: 250-500 mg daily; take with food.

Children's Dose
Acetaminophen:

Age	Wgt	325mg tab	80mg tab or 1/2 tsp 160mg liquid
4-5	36-48lb	3/4	3
6-8	48-59lb	1	4
9/10	60-71lb	1-1/4	5
11/12	72-95lb	1-1/2	6

Aspirin: **NOT RECOMMENDED FOR CHILDREN.**
Ibuprofen: 4.5 mg per pound of body weight, maximum = 15 mg per day; take with food.
Naproxen: 4.5 mg per pound of body weight, maximum = 15 mg per day; take with food.

Referencers on Page 43

23

BLISTERS

Caused by friction from skin being rubbed by an ill-fitting shoe, a seam or fold in a sock, or holding a racquet or ski pole. Cover vulnerable regions with tape, bandages, moleskin, or gloves.

Immediate Attention

1. Lubricate pre-blister irritation ("hot spot") with petroleum jelly; cover with gauze or moleskin; possibly cool with ice.

2. Do not pick or pull at a blister. Use a moleskin doughnut pad until healed.

3. Wash a broken blister frequently with soap and warm water and cover it with a sterile dressing; trim ragged edges with a sterile scissors.

Consult a physician IF...

• signs of infection appear: pus oozing from the blistered region, redness, pain, or swelling.

Referencers on Page 42

BRUISE (*Contusion*)

A bruise (*contusion*) is the result of damaged muscle tissue and blood vessels from a blow to some part of the body.

Immediate Attention

1. R.I.C.E. (rest, ice, compression, elevation).

2. Ice often during first 24 hours, less often 24-48 hours after.

3. Take acetaminophen or ibuprofen for pain (see page 23).

4. Rest the injured region until swelling and soreness subside.

5. Do not massage the injury.

Consult a physician IF...

- there is complete loss of function in the region.
- the injured region is deformed.
- pain and swelling persist for more than one week.
- an underlying bone may be injured.

References on Page 43

SUNBURN

Sunburn is due to overexposure of the skin to ultraviolet (uv) radiation. Prevention requires limiting exposure to ultraviolet radiation by covering the skin with clothes and ultraviolet absorbing lotions or sprays with SPF greater than 30.

Immediate Attention

1. Cool sunburned skin with cold compresses or cold bath (not ice). Avoid a hot shower or bath.

2. If desired for pain, acetaminophen or ibuprofen (see page 23).

3. If desired, apply lubricants to soothe the skin. Do not use butter or oils as they trap heat and cause more discomfort.

Consult a physician IF...

• blisters appear.
• nausea, vomiting, or feeling woozy occur.
• the victim is taking antibiotics.

First Aid for Sports Injuries

MOVEMENT SYSTEM INJURIES

Body movements are the result of bones being moved by muscles. Thus, many sports injuries occur to bones and muscles and the tissues that connect them.

Muscles are composed of bands of protein fibers that have the ability to shorten or "contract." When muscles contract, the bones to which they are attached move, and so do you.

Muscles are connected to bones by fibrous bands called *tendons*. Usually the fibers of a tendon and the fibers of its muscle are interwoven to form a single functional unit. Tendons do not contract as muscles do, but they can stretch, which helps flexibility. An acute (rapid) overstretching, ripping, or tearing of a muscle and possibly its associated tendon is a muscle-tendon unit *strain*. A tendon can be completely pulled away from the bone to which it is attached (called an *avulsion*). Chronic, continuous, inflammation of a tendon is *tendinitis*.

A *joint* is where two or more bones meet (*articulate*). Bones in a joint are held together by fibrous bands (different than tendons) called *ligaments*. A *sprain* is a partial or complete tearing of a ligament, which can deform (*dislocate*) or destabilize a joint.

The ends of the bones in joints are covered by an elastic material (*cartilage*) to lessen the wearing away of bone ends from friction arising from movement. Joints are surrounded by biological membranes (*bursa*) that make a lubricating fluid that allows bones to move freely. Inflammation of a bursa is *bursitis*.

Movement system injuries are either "acute," that is, occur quickly, for example, getting kicked in the leg, or they are "chronic," that is, developing over time from continual overuse, for example, tennis elbow.

More about this topic at
http://ergo84.com/fa/move.html

27

INFLAMMATION AND REPAIR

The biological response to both acute and chronic movement system injuries involves local swelling, redness, possible loss of function, and pain. This is called *inflammation*.

• Substances from damaged tissues and blood vessels promote the accumulation of fluid in the region.
• Local internal bleeding occurs but the blood eventually clots to form a hard, black-and-blue mass (*hematoma*) that may be painful and impede function.
• White blood cells accumulate in the injured region to clean away tissue debris and foreign material, bacteria, and dirt.
• Specific substances from the injured region stimulate certain nerve fibers that transmit messages to the brain, causing the sensation of pain. Pain signals the brain that something is wrong and to stop activity.

After inflammation has subsided, healing and repair can take place. Special cells (*fibroblasts*) accumulate in the injured region. They produce new fibers that knit together torn or broken fibers of muscle, tendon, or ligament. Muscle can repair in several days; tendons and ligament, several weeks.

More about this topic at
http://ergo84.com/fa/type.html

COMMON MOVEMENT SYSTEM INJURIES

Contusion
Contusion is the medical name for bruise; it is the result of a traumatic blow to the body. Contusion involves the accumulation of tissue debris, blood, and other tissue fluids that leak from damaged tissue. Normally, accumulated blood forms a clot (*hematoma*) which can sometimes be visible as a black-and-blue bruise. Immediate first aid for contusion is R.I.C.E. (see page 1); long-term care involves about two weeks of heat treatment and mild stretching.

Muscle-Tendon Strain
Acute Strain is the overstretching, ripping, or tearing of a muscle and/or its tendon. The damage can range from tearing a few fibers to complete rupture of a muscle and/or tendon.

Avulsion is complete tearing away of a muscle-tendon unit from the bone to which it is attached.

Strains tend to occur in the weakest part of a muscle-tendon unit. Strains occur because a muscle is being asked to do more than it is capable of, perhaps because it is weak from underuse or prior injury, the muscles with which it is cooperating to produce a movement are stronger, it may be fatigued, and/or it may lack sufficient water or minerals to carry out its work.

Chronic Strain results from prolonged inflammation of a muscle and/or tendon from repeated, low-grade strain. Chronic strain is characterized by local pain, point tenderness, swelling, and perhaps weakness. Chronic strain of a tendon is *tendinitis*.

Chronic strain of the lubricating sac surrounding a tendon is *tenosynovitis*. Treatment of chronic strain is rest, heat treatments, and gradual stretching. Complete healing may require several weeks.

More about this topic at
http://ergo84.com/fa/type.html

First Aid for Sports Injuries

Ligament Sprain

Sprains are partial or complete tears of ligaments that result in destabilization of a joint. *Dislocation* is when the ligamentous support of a joint is damaged such that the bones are no longer in proper alignment. R.I.C.E. is the immediate treatment for sprain. Rest, support, and heat treatments are required for complete repair, which can take several weeks. Strengthening muscles around a joint can provide protection against sprains and help stabilize a joint already weakened by prior sprain.

Fracture

A *fracture* is a break in a bone. Sometimes the break is incomplete -- the bone may be cracked. Sometimes the bone is completely parted in one or more places. If the broken ends of a bone remain within the body, the fracture is said to be *simple*. If the end of a broken bone protrudes the skin, it is said to be *compound*.

Head Injury

When the head suddenly and violently hits an object, the ground, or the side of a helmet, or when an object pierces the skull and enters brain tissue, the brain may be injured and its functioning impaired. Impact head injuries are called concussions or *traumatic brain injury* (TBI). Mild cases of TBI may result in a brief change in mental state or consciousness; severe cases may result in extended periods of unconsciousness, coma, or even death. About 500,000 sports-related head injuries occur in the United States each year.

More about this topic at
http://ergo84.com/fa/type.html

FOOT AND ANKLE INJURIES

The foot is made up of 26 bones -- 14 in the toes, five in the middle of the foot (*metatarsals*), and seven in the top and back of the foot (*tarsals*), including the ankle bone (*talus*) and heel bone (*calcaneus*).

• *Ankle sprain* is the stretching, tearing, or rupturing of the ligaments that attach the lower leg bones to the foot bones.
• *Plantar fasciitis* is soreness on the bottom of the foot ("plantar side") from overuse.
• *Stress fracture* or *fatigue fracture* is a break in one or more foot bones from continued or excessive pressure on the foot.
• *"Turf" toe* is sprain of the ligaments that connect the big toe to the rest of the foot, causing pain at the ball of the foot.
• *Exostocis* is an outgrowth of one or more of the foot bones, most often caused by poorly fitting shoes. Common sites of exostoces are the outside of the foot just below the little toe and on the heel.
• *Bunions* are tender, often painful, outgrowths on the side of the foot just below the big toe and/or little toe ("tailor's bunion"). They are usually caused by ill-fitting shoes that irritate the bone causing painful inflammation and swelling.
• *Hammer toe* is a deformation of the toes from too-short shoes.
• *Ingrown toenails* tend to occur on the big toe because that toenail grows in a spiral fashion and thus tends to grow inward. Prevention involves wearing well fitting shoes and proper nail trimming.
• *Heel* or *stone bruise* results from frequent, forceful compression of the heel, often from repetitive jumping (e.g., dancing, basketball, hurdling). Treat with R.I.C.E. and prevent/protect with padding the heel or using a heel cup.

More about this topic at
http://ergo84.com/fa/foot.html

HEAD, NECK, AND FACE INJURIES

Injuries to the head, neck, eyes, and mouth are among the most serious in sports. Head, neck, and face injuries almost always are due to collisions with other players, another part of one's own body, a ball, bat, or other piece of equipment, the ground, a fence, or a wall. Such collisions can cause brain and nerve damage, sprains of ligaments that support the vertebrae of the spine, strains of muscles in the neck, fractures of bones in the head and face, and damage to the eyes and teeth.

Concussion is brain injury caused by a traumatic blow to the head. Depending on the force of the blow, damage from a concussion can produce symptoms that are mild to severe. These include headache, dizziness, confusion, inability to answer questions quickly, poor concentration, inability to track with the eyes, nausea, vomiting, and ringing in the ears. A suspected concussion is ***always*** a reason to discontinue activity and to **consult a physician immediately**, even if symptoms abate.

Neck injuries are generally the result of impact forces. Such injuries can be highly debilitating because nerves coursing from the brain to the rest of the body pass through the neck. If a nerve is damaged, movement and sensation can be impaired. Any neck injury requires immediate medical consultation, even if symptoms abate.

"Stingers" or "burners" are painful injuries to nerves in the neck or upper torso that produce a transient burning sensation and loss of sensation in the shoulder, arm, and hand.

**More about this topic at
http://ergo84.com/fa/head.html**

KNEE INJURIES

The function of the knee is to bend. The *quadriceps* muscles ("quads") in the front of the thigh pull the lower leg toward the thigh to straighten the leg. The *hamstrings* in the back of the thigh pull the lower leg toward the butt to flex the leg at the knee.

Non-bony tissue called *cartilage* sits between the upper and lower leg bones to allow smooth rotation at the knee joint. Injury to that tissue is the "torn cartilage" so often mentioned in relation to knee injuries.

The knee is held together by ligaments that prevent excessive side-to-side and back-and-forth movements of the bones of the joint. The entire knee joint is surrounded by a membranous sac that makes a lubricating fluid. Inflammation of the sac, generally from overuse of the knee joint, is *knee bursitis*. Trauma to the knee can activate fluid-making to deal with the injury. The extra fluid, misnamed "water on the knee," can cause the knee to swell and be tender and painful.

Damage to the supporting ligaments are the most common knee injuries. One reason is that the knee's integrity depends almost entirely on support from ligaments and tendons. Another reason is that sports activity can include sudden stopping and change of direction, which puts enormous forces on the knee joint. The infamous ACL (*anterior cruciate ligament*) injury, the abbreviator of many an athletic career, is the result of a sudden twisting motion.

The kneecap (*patella*) is held in place by ligaments and tendons, which can be damaged by blows to the knee or overuse. "Jumper's knee" (*patellar tendinitis*) is caused by overuse of the patellar tendon from repeated vertical jumping (e.g., rebounding in basketball or spiking in volleyball).

More information on this topic at
http://ergo84.com/fa/knee.html

LEG INJURIES

The lower leg has two bones, the inner *tibia* and outer *fibula*. The fibula connects the knee to the foot. Contraction of muscles in the front of the lower leg pull the top of the foot toward the knee (*dorsiflexion*). Contraction of the calf muscles tips the heel and bottom of the foot downward (*plantarflexion*). Other leg muscles turn the foot inward or outward.

The upper leg has one very large bone, the *femur*. Contraction of the quadriceps muscles ("quads") in the front of the thigh straighten the leg; contraction of the hamstrings in the back of the thigh bend the leg at the knee.

Contusions (bruises) from blows to the legs are common in sports participation. Treatment = R.I.C.E. Consult a physician if swelling from blows to the front of the lower leg persists for more than two weeks (*compartment syndrome*).

Muscle cramps result from overuse and loss of minerals and fluid.

Shin splints are tenderness and pain along the inner front of the lower leg resulting from overuse.

The *Achilles tendon*, which connects the calf muscle to the heel bone, can be injured or ruptured by blows to the back of the lower leg.

.

**More about this topic at
http://ergo84.com/fa/leg.html**

First Aid for Sports Injuries

UPPER LIMB INJURIES

Injuries affecting the upper limb involve its three joints, the shoulder, elbow, and wrist. Collisions, falling, and throwing are frequent causes of damage to supporting ligaments and tendons.

Injuries to the shoulder joint include misalignment of the upper arm bone from the shoulder socket (*dislocation*) and dislodgment of the shoulder blade and collar bone (*separation*) from collision (blocking, tackling, falling). Subsequent dislocations may follow because of shoulder ligament weakness. Athletes in throwing sports risk *shoulder strain*, chronic inflammation of arm and shoulder tendons from repeated throwing motions. Overuse can also cause bursitis in the shoulder joint. Falling and overuse can damage any of the four muscle-tendon units that make up the shoulder's *rotator cuff*.

"Tennis elbow" (*lateral epicondylitis*) is the result of chronic inflammation of outside part of the elbow joint. "Pitcher's elbow" (*medial epicondylitis*) is the same type of injury on the body-side of the elbow. Tennis, badminton, and javelin throwing are also risks for elbow injury.

The ligaments of the wrist are subject to damage from falling (to break the fall), causing a *sprained wrist*.

Finger problems such as fractures, dislocations, and tendon injuries are common in baseball, basketball, and volleyball. "Baseball finger" occurs when the ball strikes the tip of the finger such that the impact tears the extensor tendon away from the bone. This puts a 30-degree bend in the end of the finger. Splinting and up to six weeks of rest are required for complete recovery and to avoid permanent deformation.

More information on this topic at
http://ergo84.com/fa/armhand.html

SKIN INJURIES AND CONDITIONS

The skin is the largest of the body's organs. Common skin conditions among athletes derive from scrapes (abrasions) and other wounds, blisters and chafing, overexposure to ultraviolet sunlight, and bacterial, viral, and fungal infection.

To lessen risks of skin conditions: Pads and skin covering for scrapes; gloves and properly fitting socks and shoes for blisters; sunscreen (SPF>30); and caution for infections.

Common skin infections include *tinea*, a fungus responsible for athlete's foot, jock itch, boils, and ringworm. *Herpesvirus* (very contagious) is responsible for cold sores and skin lesions. Allergic skin reactions (rash, itching, redness) occur from contact with offending chemicals in poison oak, sumac, ivy and other plants and products containing latex rubber, adhesives (athletic tape), and glue in sports equipment.

More about this topic at
http://ergo84.com/fa/skininj.html

HEAT AND COLD STRESS

Normal internal human body temperature is 37 degrees C. (about 98 degrees F.). Because heat always moves toward cold, the body loses heat in cold environments and absorbs heat in warm environments. Moreover, exercising muscles produce heat, which can elevate body temperature. Sweating is the evaporation of body water to rid the body of excess heat.

During exercise, replace lost body water with 4-6 ounces of tap water or dilute 100% fruit juice per 20 minutes of exercise. Sports drinks, which are artificially flavored beverages often containing carbohydrates, minerals, and electrolytes (salts), and sometimes vitamins or other nutrients, are an acceptable alternative to water and real juice. Energy drinks, which contain caffeine, **are not** recommended for children under any circumstances.

**More about this topic at
http://ergo84.com/fa/heatcold.html**

PREVENTING SPORTS INJURIES

• Listen to your body. Exertion is good. Overuse and overwork are foolish.
• Get a medical check up, especially if you are anticipating a dramatic increase in activity.
• Enjoy. Have fun. Feel good. Intense competition is unnecessary.
• Warm up and cool down.
• Strengthen muscles. Muscle weakness causes strains and overuse injuries
• Increase fitness to bolster endurance and stamina.
• Improve athletic form (obtain coaching) to reduce stress on muscles and joints.
• Stretch muscles, tendons, and ligaments.
• Focus your attention on your activity to maintain awareness of body function and environmental hazards.
• Use modern, well-functioning equipment and sports facilities.
• In extreme cold, heat, or humidity, dress appropriately, consume fluids, and be cautious.
• Rehabilitate previous injuries. Seek and adhere to professional advice.
• Match athletes by size and weight.
• Obtain adequate coaching and supervision.

**More about this topic at
http://ergo84.com/fa/prevent.html**

SPORTS INJURY FIRST AID KITS

Commercial Kits and Supplies

- *Ithaca Sports* (http://www.ithacasports.com/)
- *Cramer* (http://www.cramersportsmed.com/)
- *Lifeline* (http://www.lifelinefirstaid.com)

Self-assembled Kit
- adhesive bandages: 1-1/2"x3/8"; 3"x 3/4"; 1"x3"; 7/8"x7/8"
- butterfly bandages
- antiseptic towelettes
- alcohol cleansing pads
- antibiotic ointment ("Neosporin")
- 2"x2" sterile gauze pads
- cotton-tip applicators
- first aid tape (roll) 1/2" x 2.5 yds..
- athletic tape
- pressure bandages: 2"x 2"; 3"x 3"
- hydrogel dressings
- knee, elbow, knuckle bandages
- sterile eye wash and eye pad
- assorted safety pins
- instant ice packs
- chewable pain tablets: acetaminophen or ibuprofen
- medical grade vinyl gloves
- CPR breathing barrier
- first aid book
- elastic wrap, 2"
- hydrocortisone cream
- tweezers
- thermometer
- sunscreen
- lip balm
- moleskin (various sizes)
- pocket tissues
- emergency phone numbers
- insect repellent
- flashlight and batteries
- scissors

First Aid for Sports Injuries

REFERENCES (See also http://ergo84.com/fa/reference.html)

Page 1: R.I.C.E
• Pfeiffer, R.P. & Mangus, B.C. (2011). *Concepts of Athletic Training (6th ed.)*. Sudbury MA; JB Learning. pp 110-112.
• U.S. National Institute of Arthritis and Musculoskeletal and Skin Diseases (2009). Sports Injuries.
http://www.niams.nih.gov/Health_Info/Sports_Injuries/default.asp#ra_6.
Accessed March 11, 2012.

Page 2: Unconsciousness
• U.S. National Library of Medicine MedlinePlus (2011). Unconsciousness - first aid.
http://www.nlm.nih.gov/medlineplus/ency/article/000022.htm.
Accessed March 11, 2012.
• Fulde, G.W.O. (2009). *Emergency Medicine*. Sydney: Elsevier.

Page 3: Cardiopulmonary Resuscitation
• Cincinnati Children's Hospital (2011). CPR and Rescue Breathing.
http://www.cincinnatichildrens.org/health/a/adult-cpr/. Accessed March 7, 2011.
• U.S. National Library of Medicine MedlinePlus (2011). CPR.
http://www.nlm.nih.gov/medlineplus/cpr.html Accessed March 12, 2012.

Pages 4: Breathing Problem
• U.S. National Library of Medicine MedlinePlus (2011): CPR - Adult.
http://www.nlm.nih.gov/medlineplus/ency/article/000013.htm. Accessed March 6, 2012.
• U.S. National Library of Medicine MedlinePlus (2011): CPR - Child 1-8 Years. http://www.nlm.nih.gov/medlineplus/ency/article/000012.htm.
Accessed March 6, 2012.

Page 6: Serious Bleeding
• U.S. National Library of Medicine MedlinePlus (2011). Bleeding.
http://www.nlm.nih.gov/medlineplus/ency/article/000045.htm Accessed March 6, 2012.
• Jones, T.R. (2011). Wound Care. In C. Keith Stone & Roger L. Humphries, *Current Diagnosis and Treatment: Emergency Medicine (7th Ed.)*. NY: McGraw-Hill.

Pages 7 and 9: Cuts (Lacerations) and Punctures
• U.S. National Library of Medicine Medline Plus (2011). Cuts and puncture wounds. http://www.nlm.nih.gov/medlineplus/ency/article/000043.htm.
Accessed March 6, 2012.
• The Merck Manual for Healthcare Professionals (2011), Lacerations.
http://www.merckmanuals.com/professional/injuries_poisoning/lacerations/lacerations.html?qt=cuts%20and%20scrapes&sc=&alt=sh. Accessed Sept. 15, 2011.

First Aid for Sports Injuries

Page 8: Nosebleed
• Mayo Clinic (2011). Nosebleeds: First aid.
http://www.mayoclinic.com/health/first-aid-nosebleeds/HQ00105. Accessed
March 6, 2012.
• American Academy of Otolaryngology - Head and Neck Surgery (2011).
Nosebleeds. http://www.entnet.org/HealthInformation/Nosebleeds.cfm.
Accessed March 6, 2012.

Page 10: Scrape (Abrasion)
• U.S. National Library of Medicine MedlinePlus (2011). Wounds.
http://www.nlm.nih.gov/medlineplus/wounds.html. Accessed March 6, 2012.
• American Academy of Family Physicians (2010). First Aid: Scrapes.
http://familydoctor.org/familydoctor/en/prevention-wellness/staying-
healthy/first-aid/first-aid-cuts-scrapes-and-stitches.printerview.all.html.
Accessed March 6, 2012.

Page 11: Dental Injuries
• Pfeiffer, R.P. & Mangus, B.C. (2011). *Concepts of Athletic Training (6th ed.)*.
Sudbury MA; JB Learning. pp 136-138.
• American Academy for Sports Dentistry (2010). Emergency Treatment of
Athletic Dental Injuries.
http://academyforsportsdentistry.org/Resources/TreatmentCards/tabid/70/Defau
lt.aspx Accessed March 7, 2011.

Page 12: Eye Injuries
• American Academy of Ophthalmology (2012). Care and Treatment
Recommendations for Eye Injury.
http://www.geteyesmart.org/eyesmart/living/eye-injuries-care-treatment.cfm.
Accessed March 7, 2012.
• New York University Medical Center (2012). Eye Contusion.
http://pediatrics.med.nyu.edu/conditions-we-treat/conditions/eye-contusion.
Accessed March 12, 2012.

Page 13: Head and Neck Injuries
• Pfeiffer, R.P. & Mangus, B.C. (2011). *Concepts of Athletic Training (6th ed.)*.
Sudbury MA; JB Learning. ppg 120-124.
• U.S. National Library of Medicine MedlinePlus (2011): Head Injury.
http://www.nlm.nih.gov/medlineplus/ency/article/000028.htm. Accessed March
7, 2012.

Page 14: Genital Injuries
• U.S. National Library of Medicine PubMed Health (2011). Genital Injury.
http://www.ncbi.nlm.nih.gov/pubmedhealth/PMH0001111/
Accessed March 9, 2012.
• U.S. National Library of Medicine MedlinePlus (2011): Genital Injury.
http://www.nlm.nih.gov/medlineplus/ency/article/000044..htm. Accessed
March 8, 2012.

First Aid for Sports Injuries

Page 15: Cold Stress
• Wilmore, J.H. et al. (2008). *Physiology of Sport and Exercise*. (4th Ed.): Champaign, IL: Human Kinetics. pg. 275.
• International Association of Athletic Federations (2011). Environmental factors influencing human performance. Accessed March 6, 2012. http://www.iaaf.org/medical/manual/index.html.

Page 16; Frostbite
• Wilmore, J.H. et al. (2008). *Physiology of Sport and Exercise*. (4th Ed.): Champaign, IL: Human Kinetics. pg. 275.
• International Association of Athletic Federations (2011). Environmental factors influencing human performance.
http://www.iaaf.org/medical/manual/index.html

Page 17: Heat Stress
• University of Maryland Medical School (2011). Heat Exhaustion.
http://www.umm.edu/altmed/articles/heat-exhaustion-000075.htm. Accessed March 10, 2012.
• International Association of Athletic Federations (2011). Environmental factors influencing human performance.
http://www.iaaf.org/medical/manual/index.html. Accessed March 6, 2012.

Page 18: Heat Stroke
• Mayo Clinic (2011). Heat stroke. http://www.mayoclinic.com/health/heat-stroke/DS01025. Accessed October 7, 2011.
• National Athletic Trainers Association (2003). Parents and coaches guide to dehydration and other heat illnesses in children.
http://www.nata.org/health-issues/heat-illness. Accessed October 7, 2011.

Page 19: Broken Bone
• Mayo Clinic (2011). Fracture (broken bones): First Aid.
http://www.mayoclinic.com/print/first-aid-fractures/FA00058/METHOD=print. Accessed March 10, 2012.
• U.S. National Library of Medicine MedlinePlus (2011). Fractures.
http://www.nlm.nih.gov/medlineplus/fractures.html#cat5. Accessed March 11, 2012.

Page 20: Muscle Cramp
• American Academy of Orthopaedic Surgeons (2011). Muscle cramp.
http://orthoinfo.aaos.org/topic.cfm?topic=A00200. Accessed March 10, 2012.
• U.S. National Library of Medicine MedlinePlus (2011). Muscle Cramps.
http://www.nlm.nih.gov/medlineplus/musclecramps.html. Accessed March 11, 2012.

Page 21: Muscle Pull (Strain).
• U.S. National Library of Medicine MedlinePlus (2011). Muscle strain.
http://www.nlm.nih.gov/medlineplus/ency/article/002116.htm. Accessed March 11, 2012.
• U.S. National Institute of Arthritis and Musculoskeletal and Skin Diseases (2009). Sprains and Strains.
http://www.niams.nih.gov/Health_Info/Sprains_Strains/default.asp#strain_g. Accessed March 11, 2012.

First Aid for Sports Injuries

Page 22: Sprain
• Mayo Clinic (2010). Sprain: First aid.
http://www.mayoclinic.com/health/first-aid-sprain/FA00016. Accessed March 12, 2012.
• U.S. National Institute of Arthritis and Musculoskeletal and Skin Diseases (2009). Sprains and Strains.
http://www.niams.nih.gov/Health_Info/Sprains_Strains/default.asp#strain_g. Accessed March 11, 2012.

Page 23: Pain
• Mayo Clinic (2011). Acetaminophen and children.
http://www.mayoclinic.com/print/acetaminophen/HO00002/METHOD=print. Accessed March 12, 2012.
• American Academy of Family Physicians (2012). Pain Relievers: Understanding Your OTC Options.
http://familydoctor.org/familydoctor/en/drugs-procedures-devices/over-the-counter/pain-relievers-understanding-your-otc-options.html. Accessed March 12, 2012.

Page 24: Blisters
• Johns Hopkins Medicine (2012). Blisters.
http://www.hopkinsmedicine.org/healthlibrary/printv.aspx?d=85,P00262. Accessed March 12, 2012.
• Richie, D. (June, 2010). How to manage friction blisters. *Podiatry Today.* http://www.podiatrytoday.com/how-to-manage-friction-blisters. Accessed March 12, 2012.

Page 25: Bruise (Contusion)
• American Academy of Orthopaedic Surgeons (2007). Muscle Contusion (Bruise). http://orthoinfo.aaos.org/topic.cfm?topic=A00341&return_link=0. Accessed March 12, 2012.
• Mayo Clinic (2011). Bruise: First aid.
http://www.mayoclinic.com/health/first-aid-bruise/FA00039. Accessed March 12, 2012.

Page 26: Sunburn
• Children's Hospital of Orange County (2012). Sunburn.
http://chocchildrens.org/healthlibrary/topic.cfm?PageID=P01929. Accessed March 11, 2012.
• U.S. National Library of Medicine MedlinePlus (2011). Sun exposure.
http://www.nlm.nih.gov/medlineplus/sunexposure.html.
Accessed March 11, 2012.

First Aid for Sports Injuries

General References

Pfeiffer, R.P. & Mangus, B.C. (2011). *Concepts of Athletic Training (6th ed.)*. Sudbury MA; JB Learning.

American College of Sports Medicine
http://www.acsm.org/access-public-information/brochures-fact-sheets/fact-sheets.

U.S. National Library of Medicine MedlinePlus. (2011). Sports Injuries (2011). http://www.nlm.nih.gov/medlineplus/sportsinjuries.html.

U.S. National Institutes of Health (2011). Sports Injuries. http://www.niams.nih.gov/Health_Info/Sports_Injuries/default.asp.

Mayo Clinic on First Aid (2011). http://www.mayoclinic.com/health/FirstAidIndex/FirstAidIndex.

EMERGENCY CONTACT NUMBERS

Fire Rescue/EMT_____

Hospital _____

Police _____

Doctor Name_____

Contact _____

Doctor Name _____

Contact _____

Dentist Name_____

Contact _____

Orthodontist Name _____

Contact _____

Others

Name _____

Contact: _____

Name _____

Contact _____

Name _____

Contact _____

Add these Contacts to your cell phone

First Aid for Sports Injuries Digital Edition
for
Smart Phones and Tablets

First Aid
for
Sports
Injuries

Fast access to helpful information when someone is injured at practice, during competition, working out, and at recreational play.

More info:
***First Aid for Sports Injuries* Web site**
http://ergo84.com/fa/